better nutrition *magazine* presents

DENTAL HEALTH

by JOHN PELDYAK, DMD

better nutrition healthy living guide

Published by:
Active Interest Media, Inc.
300 N. Continental Blvd., Suite 650
El Segundo, CA 90245

This booklet is part of the *Better Nutrition Healthy Living Guide* series. For more information, visit www.betternutrition.com. Better Nutrition magazine is available at fine natural health stores throughout the United States. Design by Aline Design: Bellingham, Wash.

DENTAL HEALTH

CONTENTS

better nutrition healthy living guide

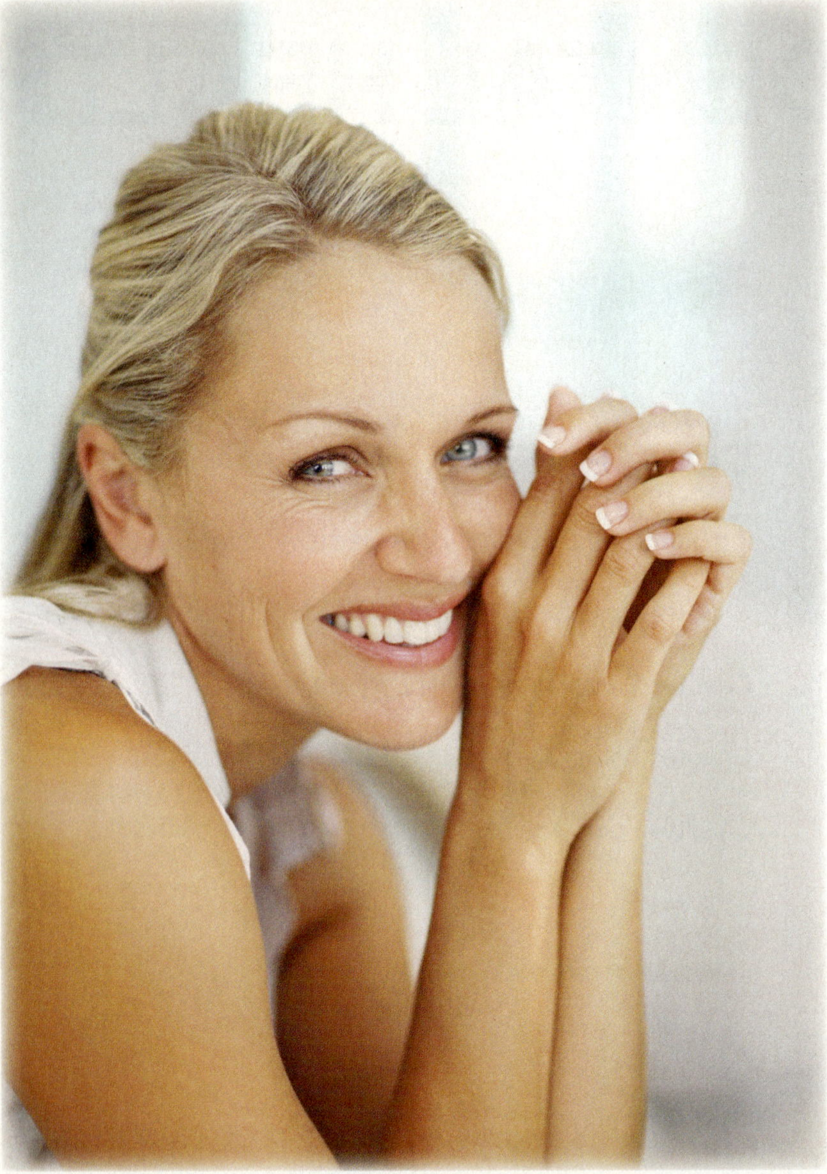

"There is not one thing in preventive medicine as important as oral hygiene and the preservation of the teeth."

–Sir William Osler

Introduction

Enemies of a Healthy Smile

Brush, floss, rinse: three simple steps that are supposed to keep our teeth and gums healthy for a lifetime. Yet, reality paints a far different picture. According to the National Institutes of Health, most adults show signs of both tooth decay and periodontal disease. It's so serious that two-thirds of middle aged Americans have lost at least one tooth to a cavity—technically known as dental caries—or to gum disease. And the problem just grows worse as people get older. Among those over 60, one-fourth have lost all of their teeth to decay. This means that untreated periodontal disease is responsible for more lost teeth than cavities, particularly in the aged.

Among children, decay is the most prevalent chronic disease of childhood. And it can start as young as age 2. The Centers for Disease Control and Prevention report that tooth decay affects more than one-fourth of U.S. children aged 2 to 5 and half of those between the ages of 12 and 15. By children reach their late teens (age 16 to 19), 68 percent have experienced one or more dental caries.

The Causes of Poor Oral Health

These statistics can be attributed to a number of factors. Some, like advancing age, the genes you are born with, diseases like diabetes, dry mouth, and even fluctuating hormones, are beyond your control. But the most common causes of tooth decay and periodontal disease stem from lifestyle choices, including the following.

- **A high sugar diet.** It's no secret that the frequent consumption of sweets contributes to tooth decay. Eating a diet containing lots of sugar and starch increases the risk of cavities. Sticky foods like raisins, cookies, or even plain white bread can be a particular problem because they are more likely to remain on the surface of the teeth. When this occurs, the sugar will react with the bacteria in your mouth and produce harmful acids. Frequent snacking also increases the amount of time that these acids are in contact with the teeth. In fact, every time you eat or drink anything sugary, your teeth are under acid attack for up to one hour. This is why it is important to limit sweets to mealtimes only, which limits the amount of time your mouth is at risk.

- **Poor dental hygiene habits.** Too often, we give our teeth a lick and a promise, or sometimes forget to brush at all. But poor dental hygiene is the No. 1 way we undermine healthy teeth. Dull, yellowed teeth, cavities, and gum disease are all caused by the buildup of plaque, a sticky substance that forms when mucus, food particles, and bacteria interact with saliva. If plaque isn't removed from teeth it will eventually mineralize into tartar, a hard substance that is extremely difficult to get rid of. That is why it is critical to brush and floss at least twice each day.
- **Smoking.** Smoking cigarettes can cause a variety of serious, even life-threatening diseases like emphysema, heart disease, stroke, and cancer. But few people realize that tobacco use can also lead to both tooth decay and periodontal disease. Smoking, and even smokeless tobacco, increases the buildup of plaque and tartar on the teeth. It can also lead to gum disease by affecting the attachment of bone and soft tissue to your teeth. More specifically, smoking appears to interfere with the normal function of gum tissue cells. This makes smokers more susceptible to infections like periodontal disease. It also impairs blood flow to the gums, which may affect wound healing. What's more, smoking increases one's risk of developing oral cancer.

The good news is that you don't need to become one of the statistics. Adopting a healthy lifestyle and practicing good oral hygiene on a daily basis can help keep your teeth and gums healthy. But there's even more you can do. Adding xylitol—a naturally occurring sweetener that tastes like sugar—to the equation can mean the difference between a dazzling smile and a mouthful of trouble. But before we explore this amazing tooth-preserving compound that comes from fruits and vegetables, let's take a closer look at what's going on in your mouth.

Chapter One
Oral Health 101

The mouth is undoubtedly one of the most utilized areas of the body. We use it to speak, eat, breathe, and even express our feelings. Yet, unless there's a problem, we don't give much thought to what's behind our lips. But your mouth (known in medicine as the oral cavity) is a wonderfully designed machine with many different parts that operate all together to keep you alive, healthy, and happy.

Behind Your Smile

Your mouth is made up of several parts, including the teeth, gingiva (gums), tongue, palate, cheeks, lips, and the floor of your mouth. All of these components, except for the teeth, are lined by mucous membranes. Here is a quick primer of what each of these parts does:

- The gingiva is the soft tissue that covers the bone holding your teeth in place. The gingiva surrounds the teeth and covers the jawbone, creating a protective barrier.
- The tongue is a muscular organ responsible for taste. It also plays a critical role in the ability to chew, digest, swallow, and speak.
- The palate, commonly known as the roof of the mouth, is divided into the hard palate and the soft palate. The hard palate is the solid, immovable area that attaches to the teeth and gums, forming an arch. The soft palate, which is located toward the back of the throat, is the flexible area of the mouth in which the gag reflex occurs.
- The cheeks form the sides of the mouth and continue along the front of the face to the lips. The cheeks are made up of subcutaneous fat, with the outside layer covered by skin and the inside consisting of a mucous membrane. The cheek muscles (the buccinators) are responsible for our ability to smile, swallow, and keep food in our mouths when we eat.
- The floor of the mouth is formed by mucous membranes. These membranes extend inward from both sides of the lower jawbone and from the tongue to the gum line, forming a crescent shape. Within the floor of the mouth are glands, portions of the muscles of the tongue, and nerves.

- The lips are the soft and pliable fleshy tissue that connects to the front area of the cheeks. The outside of the lips is covered by skin. The gingiva attaches to the part of the lips inside the mouth that is covered by the mucous membrane. Blood vessels close to the surface of the skin give lips their red color. In addition to helping us speak, the lips help keep food between the top and bottom teeth while also guiding it through the mouth.

Your Teeth

Your teeth are arranged in two arches—one arch in the upper jaw and one in the lower. Children have 20 primary, or baby, teeth and begin to develop their first permanent teeth by age 6. Adults normally have 32 permanent teeth. With proper care, these permanent teeth will last a lifetime.

There are several types of permanent teeth from front to back: incisors, canines, premolars, and molars. Each tooth is made up of the area you can see past the gum line—an area known as the anatomical crown—and several other parts that you can't see. Below the crown is the root, which is the part of the tooth that pushes into the upper (maxilla) or lower (mandible) jawbone.

Each tooth has several layers, including the enamel, dentin, and pulp. Just beneath the enamel (which covers the crown) and the cementum (which covers the root) is the dentin, the hard inner layer of the tooth. The pulp is located beneath the dentin at the core of the tooth. It contains blood vessels, nerves, and connective tissue and is surrounded by the gums to hold the teeth in place.

Proper dental care—including a nourishing diet, frequent cleaning, and regular checkups—is essential to maintaining a healthy mouth and keeping tooth decay and gum disease at bay. Unfortunately, that isn't the norm for most people as they age. Instead of a dazzling smile, they find themselves in the dentist's chair facing fillings, root canals, extractions, or worse.

When Things Go Wrong

The absence of even one tooth can cause problems with digestion, speech, and appearance. Poor diet, hit-or-miss dental care, and bad habits like smoking can undermine oral health. But, other factors can also contribute to tooth loss and periodontal disease.

People with diabetes are more prone to dental caries. When diabetes is not well-controlled, high blood sugar levels in saliva may help bacteria

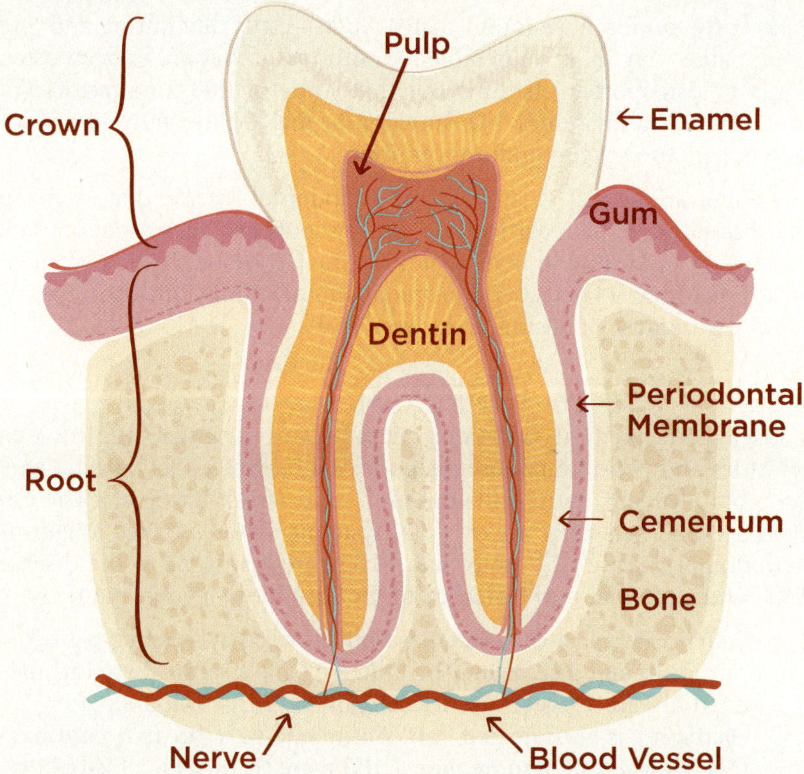

thrive. Even when blood sugar levels are adequately managed, people with diabetes are at a greater risk of developing caries than the general population. One reason is that diabetics often suffer from dry mouth and, without sufficient saliva, bacteria can flourish. This was recently seen in a study that compared the oral health of 154 type 2 diabetics with 50 healthy people. Sixty-two percent of the diabetics reported chronic dry mouth. When the researchers took a closer look, they discovered that the participants who didn't produce enough saliva had significantly higher numbers of *Streptococcus mutans* (S. mutans), the bacteria that causes tooth decay.

People with uncontrolled diabetes are also at greater risk of periodontal disease. Because diabetes reduces the body's resistance to infection, the gums are among the tissues likely to be affected. When periodontal disease develops in someone with uncontrolled diabetes, it is often more severe and causes more tooth loss than in someone who has good control of his diabetes.

Recently, studies have found that women—especially during and after menopause—are more vulnerable to tooth loss if they suffer from osteopenia or osteoporosis. It turns out that some of the same factors that undermine healthy bones, like smoking or the overconsumption of soft drinks, can also set you up for tooth loss.

Women are also at greater risk of periodontal disease due to changing hormone levels, particularly during puberty, menstruation, and pregnancy. According to investigators at the Cleveland Clinic's Women's Health Institute, 44 percent of postmenopausal women can also suffer the same fate because of declining estrogen levels.

Healthy Mouth, Healthy You

Just as some medical conditions can make you more susceptible to dental caries and periodontal disease, poor oral health can let bacteria enter your bloodstream, cause inflammation, and wreak havoc elsewhere in your body. In fact, there are over 100 systemic diseases linked to chronic periodontal disease and tooth decay. Here are just some of the diseases and conditions that may be linked to the condition of your mouth:

- **Cardiovascular disease.** Research shows that several types of cardiovascular disease may be linked to oral health. These include heart disease, clogged arteries, and stroke. Periodontal disease, even if it has been treated, can continue to be a threat. According to a clinical trial of more than 1,100 men, those with a history of periodontal disease had a higher risk of having a stroke than those who had never developed gum disease.
- **Pregnancy and birth.** Gum disease has been linked to premature birth and low-birthweight babies. This is why it's vital to maintain excellent oral health before you get pregnant and during your pregnancy.
- **Diabetes.** Diabetes increases your risk of gum disease, cavities, tooth loss, dry mouth, and a variety of oral infections. Conversely, poor oral health can make your diabetes more difficult to control. Infections and subsequent inflammation may cause your blood sugar to rise and require more insulin to keep it under control.
- **HIV/AIDS.** Oral problems are very common with HIV/AIDS. Symptoms can include ulcers, dry mouth, and related painful mucosal lesions. Mouth problems are caused by fungal, viral, or bacterial infections and, in some cases, one of the first signs of AIDS may be severe gum infection. Persistent white spots or unusual lesions may develop on the tongue or in the mouth.

- **Osteoporosis.** The first stages of bone loss may show up around your teeth. Systemic loss of bone density in osteoporosis, including bone in the jaw, may create a condition in which the bone supporting your teeth is increasingly susceptible to infectious destruction. Your dentist may be able to spot this on a routine clinical examination or with dental X-rays.
- **Cancer.** Recent evidence from Harvard has found that men with poor oral health were 64 percent more likely to develop pancreatic cancer. Another study conducted at Imperial College London in the United Kingdom discovered that, compared to men with healthy gums, men with a history of gum disease had a 36 percent increased risk of lung cancer, a 49 percent hike in risk of kidney cancer, and a 30 percent increased risk of white blood cell cancers. In addition, men who had fewer teeth at the beginning of the study had a 70 percent increased risk of developing lung cancer, compared with men who had 25 to 32 teeth. While much of this research is in the early stages, scientists think that chronic infection in the mouth can trigger inflammation throughout the body. This, in turn, may spark a chemical process in the body that results in high levels of cancer-causing compounds known as nitrosamines.
- **Other conditions.** Many other conditions may make their presence known in your mouth before you even know that anything is wrong. These may include Sjogren's syndrome, eating disorders, syphilis, gonorrhea, and substance abuse.

While basic hygiene can help protect your smile and keep these health problems from developing, there is an easy, remarkably effective addition you can make to your daily routine that will give you optimal protection against tooth decay. It's a natural sugar known as xylitol.

Chapter Two
The Xylitol Difference

A sugar that promotes healthy teeth? It may sound a bit far-fetched, but it's true. Xylitol is a white crystalline sugar alcohol that looks and tastes just like the sugar in your sugar bowl. Xylitol is found naturally in many fruits and vegetables like berries, plums, lettuce, and mushrooms. But, instead of promoting tooth decay, xylitol can actually help prevent it.

What makes xylitol so special? While at first glance this natural substance might be mistaken for refined sugar, it has 40 percent fewer calories than sugar. But it's xylitol's health benefits that make this natural sweetener so remarkable. Xylitol

- helps prevent tooth decay;
- reduces plaque formation on teeth;
- blocks the acids that demineralize tooth enamel;
- helps repair damaged enamel;
- halts the growth of specific types of acid-producing bacteria linked to tooth decay;
- helps reduce gingival inflammation;
- relieves dry mouth;
- helps maintain upper-respiratory health and thwarts ear infections by combating bacteria in the nasopharynx;
- may help prevent osteoporosis;
- does not trigger an insulin reaction in the body, making it useful for diabetics and those who are hypogloycemic;
- has a low rating on the glycemic index (7); and
- is safe for all ages.

The Molecular Difference

According to Professor Kauko Mäkinen of the Institute of Dentistry in Finland and a pioneer in xylitol research, the chemical profile of xylitol isn't like other natural sweeteners. He notes in a recent publication, *Xylitol: An Amazing Discovery for Health*, that many of these naturally occurring sugar substitutes are part of a family of sugar alcohols called polyols. Polyols (like sorbitol, mannitol, maltitol, and other sweeteners that end in "-ol") are considered carbohydrates closely related to sugars (sweeteners that generally end in "-ose"), but tend to be less reactive and lower in calories.

What makes xylitol different from other sweeteners? Most of our dietary carbohydrates (sugars and polyols) are based on a 6-carbon monosaccharide unit like fructose (fruit sugar) and glucose (aka d-glucose, dextrose, blood sugar). Saccharide units can be linked together into disaccharides such as sucrose (common table sugar that is glucose and fructose bonded together), or polysaccharides that can have hundreds of saccharides connected (starch is composed of long strings of 6-carbon glucose units). Instead of the six carbon atoms found in other sweeteners, xylitol contains only five. This unique 5-carbon sugar alcohol structure is very stable and does not link together with other sugars.

The stable five-carbon architecture gives xylitol some unique properties. Unlike sugars (and to a lesser extent other polyols), xylitol is not a good food source for bacteria and yeast. Sugars promote tooth decay. But xylitol acts as the natural dental antidote for sugar, blocking its harmful effects and building protective factors.

Xylitol was discovered by German and French scientists simultaneously in 1890. By the 1930s, it had been purified, but, this unique sweetener wasn't used commercially until World War II when it was extracted from birch trees in Finland in response to a shortage of sugar. It was also during

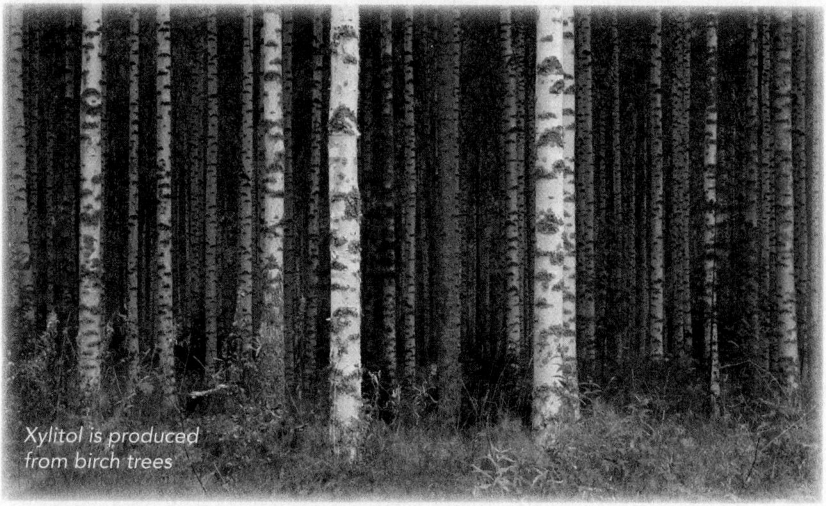

Xylitol is produced from birch trees

this time that researchers discovered xylitol's ability to metabolize in the body without using insulin. By the early 1960s, xylitol was being used in Germany, Switzerland, the Soviet Union, and Japan as a premium sweetener for people with diabetes. It also found its way into IV solutions as an energy source for patients with impaired glucose tolerance and insulin resistance. Xylitol was approved by the U.S. Food and Drug Administration in 1963 for special dietary purposes.

Oddly enough, xylitol's most important health benefit—its ability to improve dental health—wasn't fully appreciated until the 1970s. After initial findings hinted at xylitol's remarkable ability to prevent tooth decay, long-term clinical trials were launched. In one study, all accessible sugar was removed from the diet and replaced with xylitol. The volunteers were closely monitored for overall health, and a dramatic reduction in tooth decay was noted.

A parallel group obtained similar results by using only small amounts of xylitol in chewing gum after meals. The first xylitol chewing gum hit the market in Finland and became an immediate success. Since then, several dental and medical associations throughout the world have endorsed its use.

Xylitol looks, feels, and tastes exactly like sugar and leaves no unpleasant aftertaste. It can replace equal amounts of sugar in cooking or baking and can be used as a sweetener for beverages. It is also included as an ingredient in chewing gum, mints, and candy, as well as toothpastes, mouthwashes, and nasal sprays.

A Safe Sugar Alternative

Not only does xylitol possess a wealth of healthy benefits, it is also safe. A scientific committee of the United Nations' World Health Organization and Food and Agriculture Organization (the Joint Expert Committee on Food Additives) announced that xylitol, at levels up to 90 grams per day, is a safe sweetener for foods. Today, dentists around the world recommend its use in both adults and children as a convenient and nontoxic way to enhance oral health. Studies show that even infants can safely benefit from xylitol.

About one-third of the xylitol that is consumed is absorbed in the liver. The other two-thirds travels to the intestinal tract where it is broken down by gut bacteria into short-chain fatty acids such as butarate, which can improve overall colon health. While most people don't experience any side effects, people who are sensitive to xylitol may initially experience loose stools or slight abdominal cramping when they ingest too much of it, particularly on an empty stomach. But, since the body itself makes

While you might think that enamel would protect teeth from damage, it's no match for the decay-causing acid produced by S. mutans.

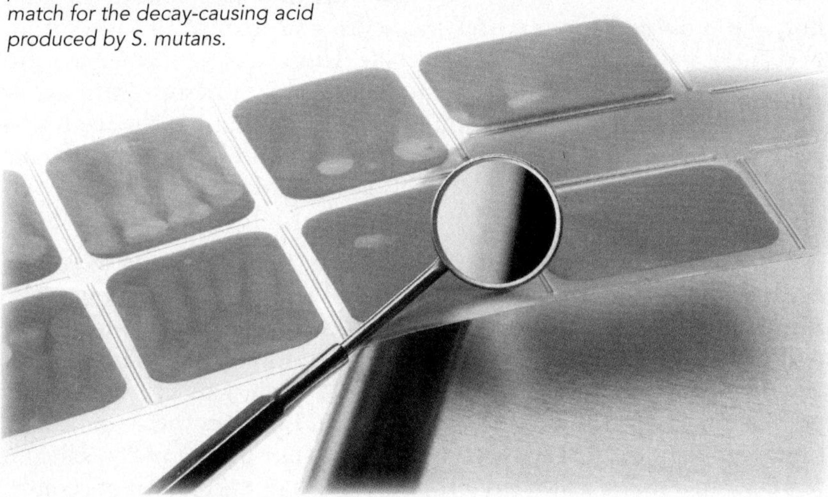

xylitol—as well as the enzymes to break it down—larger amounts can be tolerated within a few days or weeks as the body's enzymatic activity adjusts to a higher intake.

Streptococcus Mutans' Natural Foe

No matter how often we brush, all of us have bacteria flourishing in our mouths. The mouth is the perfect place for bacteria. It's dark, warm, and wet. In fact, more than 600 different groups of bacteria call the human mouth home. While most of these bacteria are perfectly harmless, one type—*Streptococcus mutans* (S. mutans)—has been directly linked to tooth decay.

What makes S. mutans so treacherous to our teeth? When these micro-organisms feed on the carbohydrates and sugars we eat, they metabolize these foods by fermenting them. This, in turn, triggers the secretion of lactic acid onto the hard enamel surface of teeth. While you might think that enamel would protect teeth from damage, it's no match for the decay-causing acid produced by S. mutans. So, even though tooth enamel is the hardest substance in the body, ongoing exposure to this corrosive acid gradually dissolves the enamel, leaving teeth vulnerable to decay.

Left alone, S. mutans will happily multiply in this acidic environment, combining with leftover sugar debris to form a sticky biofilm known as plaque that adheres to the teeth. If plaque isn't removed on a daily basis, it accumulates. This accumulation—which occurs most frequently between teeth and at or under the gum line—shelters more acid germs and can harden into tartar. When plaque accumulates beneath the gum line, the buildup of tartar, bacteria, acids, and toxins can cause irritation and inflammation of the gum tissue. This can lead to gingivitis and periodontal disease. Continued plaque accumulation can contribute to structural damage of the teeth and the bone supporting the teeth and gums. And, as we've discussed, the resulting tooth and gum problems that stem from poor oral health can also contribute to other health complications as well.

While S. mutans may appear tough to defeat, xylitol makes it look easy. Because of its five-carbon structure, xylitol cannot be metabolized by S. mutans. This reduces the amount of acid that is produced in the mouth and essentially "starves" and weakens the harmful acid bacteria. Xylitol also helps prevent plaque from adhering to teeth, which helps to stop demineralization before it even begins; xylitol reduces the acidic effects of dental plaque. The unique structure of xylitol helps to keep calcium available in a useful form. Not only does this halt the erosion of enamel, it also encourages remineralization. Because of its capacity to thwart bacteria and remineralize enamel, xylitol has the uncanny ability to arrest and actually reverse tooth decay, at least in the early stages. This effect is long-lasting and possibly permanent.

Hundreds of studies and clinical trials have verified these extraordinary effects. But, as you will see in the next chapter, you won't get xylitol's benefits by simply popping a piece of xylitol gum every now and again. The secret to its effectiveness is frequent repeated use on a daily basis.

Chapter Three

Caring For Your Teeth

As a dentist, I've seen much tooth decay during my years of practice—and much of it could have been prevented if my patients had known about xylitol. Used four to five times per day, xylitol can help keep tooth decay from occurring—but only if it is used as part of a daily oral hygiene program. I often advise my patients to use a comprehensive, high-quality oral system like Xlear's Spry Dental Defense System. I've found that this system provides effective levels of xylitol in a range of convenient and enjoyable products that can be used throughout the day.

Brush Away Dental Problems

Brushing properly can mean the difference between a dazzling smile and a mouthful of plaque. I recommend brushing morning and night, preferably after eating. Yet, many people don't brush correctly. Proper brushing takes at least two minutes, but most of us don't come close to brushing that long. Try timing yourself until you can accurately estimate the time it takes to clean your teeth.

Use a toothbrush with soft, nylon, round-ended bristles that will not scratch and irritate teeth or damage gums. Small-headed toothbrushes are also preferable to large ones, since they can better reach all areas of the mouth, including those hard-to-reach back teeth. Apply a pea-sized amount of a xylitol toothpaste to the brush. (Studies suggest that using a toothpaste like Spry Fluoride Toothpaste that contains both xylitol and fluoride not only neutralizes harmful S. mutans bacteria, it may enhance remineralization.) Then use short, gentle strokes, paying extra attention to the gum line, hard-to-reach back teeth, and areas around fillings, crowns, or other restoration. Brushing often misses the sulcus—the small space between the tooth and the gum. To remedy this, hold your toothbrush at a 45 degree angle to your teeth and gums. Apply slight pressure and use a small back and forth motion so that the bristles slip into the sulcus.

Remember to replace your toothbrush every three to four months. Researchers have established that thousands of microbes grow on toothbrush bristles and handles. Most are harmless, but others can cause cold and flu viruses, the herpes virus that causes cold sores, and bacteria that can cause periodontal infections.

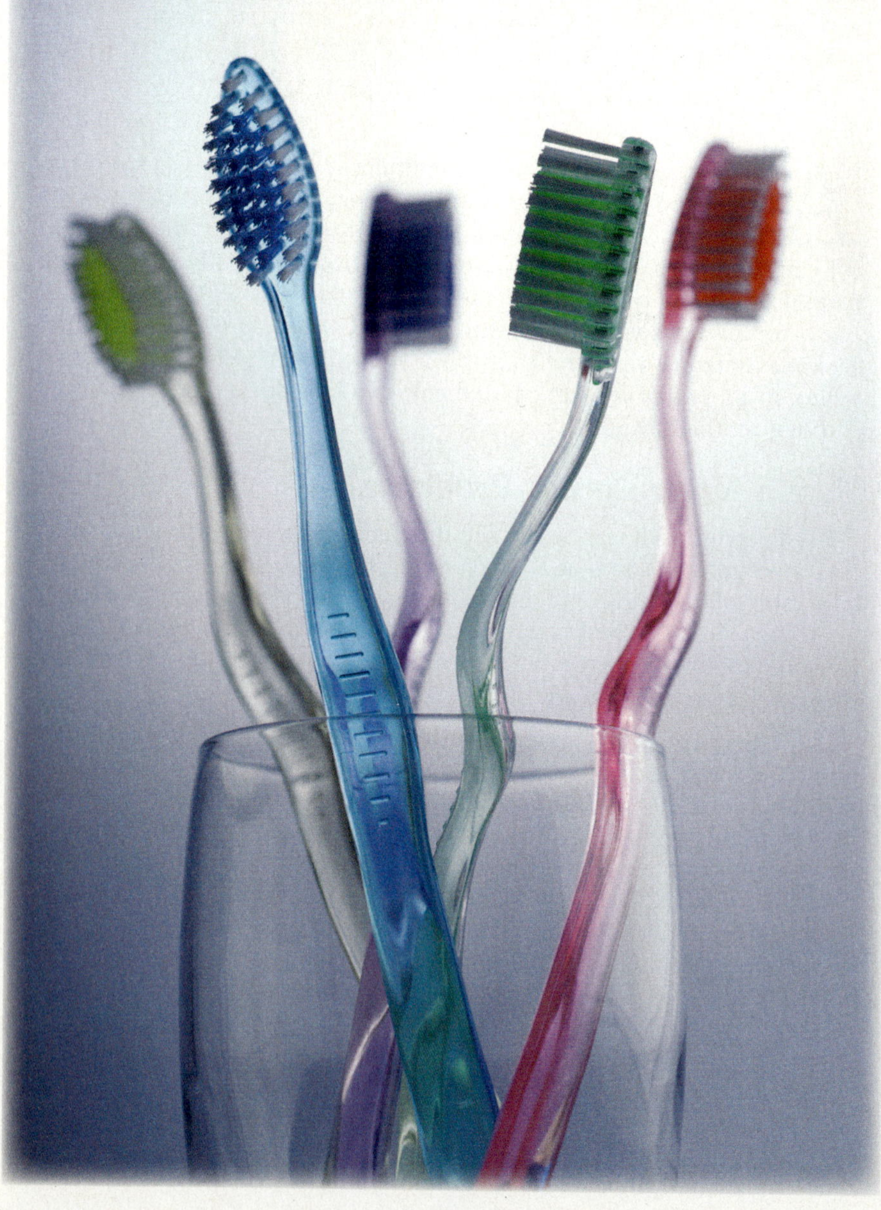

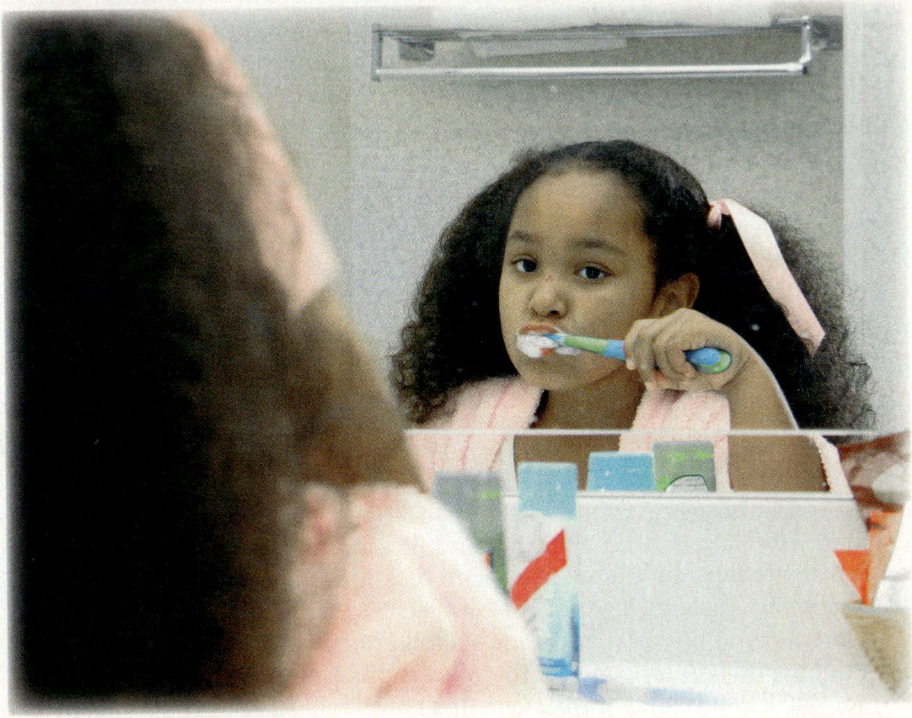

Concentrate on thoroughly cleaning each section of your mouth as follows:

- Clean the outer surfaces of your upper teeth, then your lower teeth.
- Clean the inner surfaces of your upper teeth, then your lower teeth.
- Clean all of the chewing surfaces.
- For fresher breath, be sure to brush your tongue, too.

Flossing—The Forgotten Step

No matter how frequently you brush, the bacterial plaque remaining on your teeth can only be effectively removed by thorough dental flossing at least once a day. However, according to scientific studies, it's important to floss after brushing to reduce the amount of bacteria that gets pushed into the gums while flossing.

In a study that appeared in the Journal of Periodontology, researchers compared the effects of twice daily flossing and tooth brushing versus brushing alone in 51 sets of twins, aged 12 to 21. One twin manually brushed her teeth and tongue twice a day for two weeks; the other twin was given the same instructions but with the addition of using dental floss. Before and after the study, researchers examined both groups for evidence of bleeding gums and bad breath. The results showed the group that flossed had 38 percent fewer sites that bled at the end of the study. What's more, overall gum bleeding improved by an average of 42 percent. In the brushing-only group the number of bleeding gum sites increased by nearly 4 percent.

To floss properly, wrap a piece of dental floss (I prefer the wider version called "dental tape") into a "C" shape, then scrape both sides of each tooth to snare any hidden plaque. Move the floss or tape up and down each tooth, not back and forth.

Other devices such as interdental brushes, toothpicks, and oral irrigators can also be helpful to clean between teeth. By itself, brushing is not enough.

Rinse Bacteria Goodbye

For a finishing touch, many of us reach for mouthwash in an attempt to kill the bacteria that brushing and flossing miss. But most over-the-counter brands are simply temporary breath fresheners and do nothing to specifically target the offending bacteria. To disable renegade bacteria, look for a mouthwash containing xylitol. I often use Spry Oral Rinse and recommend it to my patients. The sweet cooling effect of xylitol is a pleasant way to wash away the bacteria that contribute to bad breath, inflammation, and tooth decay.

During one clinical trial, Swedish researchers found that people who used a xylitol mouthwash not only had fewer S. mutans microorganisms in their saliva, they also lowered the amount of plaque clinging to their teeth. To get these benefits, simply swish a xylitol mouthwash around in your mouth for 30 seconds after brushing and flossing.

Protecting Children's Teeth

The first teeth generally begin to erupt around six months of age and all of the baby teeth, also called "deciduous" or "primary" teeth, are usually in by age 2. These baby teeth are important! Besides helping with chewing, swallowing, and speaking, they help to maintain proper spacing for the permanent teeth to follow.

If harmful "acid germs" such as S. mutans latch onto the enamel and establish themselves early on, these baby teeth can be susceptible to devastating, rampant tooth decay. Bacterial acids formed from frequent, prolonged exposure to sugars in juices or even milk break down vulnerable tooth surfaces. This condition is known as "Early Childhood Caries" (ECC), commonly called "baby bottle mouth." Conventional prevention advice recommends limiting these sugar exposures and putting baby to bed with only plain water in the bottle.

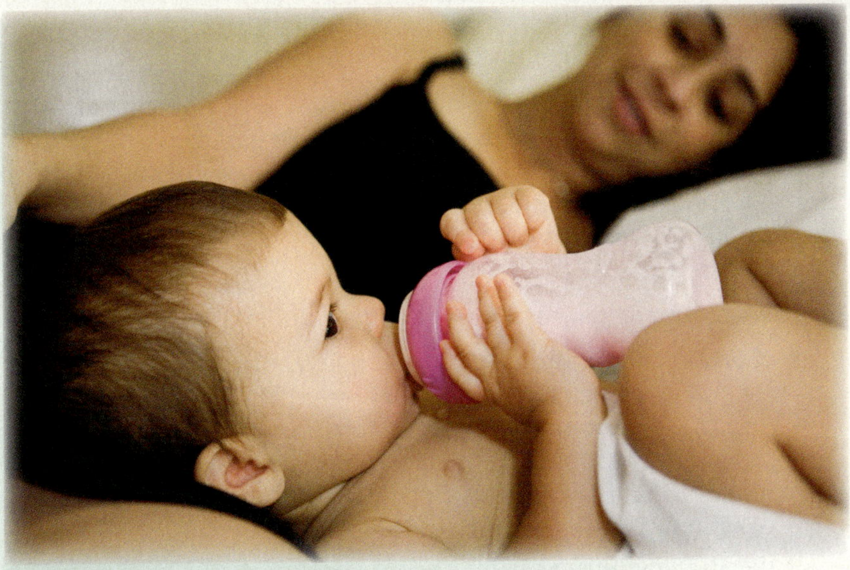

Mother-to-Child Protection

Most people are surprised to learn that dental caries is actually an infectious disease. Often decay-causing bacteria are transmitted from mother to child through everyday contact such as kissing and the tasting of food. Even mothers who have no active tooth decay can harbor enough "acid germs" to infect their babies. Early colonization by S. mutans is associated with higher decay rates, but studies show that mothers of young children can reduce the spread of S. mutans by consistently using xylitol gum and mints themselves.

One important study involving 169 pregnant women was conducted at the University of Turku, in Finland. The study was designed to establish whether routine consumption of xylitol by mothers of newborn children could prevent the transmission of S. mutans from mother to child. The expectant mothers were divided into three groups. The mothers in the test group received xylitol gum after their babies were born and instructed to chew it three to five times daily for the duration of the study. The mothers in the two control groups received either fluoride (F) or chlorhexidine (CHX) varnish applications at six, 12, and 18 months post delivery. The plaque of the children was measured once they had celebrated their second birthday. Those whose mothers hadn't used xylitol had a fivefold higher risk of S. mutans colonization compared to the children whose moms regularly used the gum. By the time the children turned 5, the xylitol group had a 70 percent lower risk of dental caries than the other two groups.

Dry Mouth

Saliva is key for keeping the mouth moist and combating harmful bacteria. Without an adequate supply of saliva, the rate of tooth decay increases rapidly. Unfortunately, many people suffer from dry mouth, a condition known in the world of dentistry as xerostomia. This can leave your mouth feeling sticky, parched, and vulnerable.

There are many causes of dry mouth, including the following.

- **Certain medications.** Dry mouth is a common side effect of many prescription and nonprescription drugs, including those used to treat depression, anxiety, pain, allergies, obesity, acne, epilepsy, hypertension, diarrhea, nausea, psychotic disorders, urinary incontinence, asthma, and Parkinson's disease. Dry mouth is also a side effect of muscle relaxants and sedatives.
- **Certain diseases and infections.** Dry mouth can be a side effect of medical conditions, including Sjögren's syndrome, HIV/AIDS, Alzheimer's disease, diabetes, anemia, cystic fibrosis, rheumatoid arthritis, hypertension, Parkinson's disease, stroke, and mumps.
- **Some medical treatments.** Damage to the salivary glands from radiation to the head and neck or chemotherapy treatments for cancer can reduce the amount of saliva produced.
- **Nerve damage.** Dry mouth can be a result of nerve damage to the head and neck area from an injury or surgery.
- **Dehydration.** Conditions that lead to dehydration, such as fever, excessive sweating, vomiting, diarrhea, blood loss, and burns can cause dry mouth.
- **Lifestyle.** Smoking or chewing tobacco can affect saliva production and aggravate dry mouth. Continuously breathing with the mouth open can also contribute to the problem.

Research shows that chewing gum can stimulate the production of saliva. But opting for a gum sweetened with xylitol offers even more benefits to people with dry mouth because it fights tooth decay and strengthens tooth enamel. Moistening the mouth with a xylitol spray also benefits people suffering from dry mouth. Plus, xylitol gum or spray is portable, easy to use, and tastes great.

While xylitol can help adults guard against tooth decay and periodontal disease, this natural sweetener is ideal for helping children avoid dental caries altogether. The perfect time to start is when a baby's teeth are about to erupt. The goal is to block the initial colonization of S. mutans and other harmful bacteria, and to optimally mineralize the new enamel. Applying a xylitol gel designed specifically for infants and toddlers is a great way to introduce your child to these benefits.

One recent double-blind, randomized trial by researchers at the University of Washington, Seattle, shows just how effective xylitol is for preventing caries in very young children. The researchers divided 100 babies between the ages of nine and 15 months into three groups. The first group was given a topical xylitol syrup by their parents twice a day. The second group received the syrup three times a day. The third group, which acted as a control group, got the xylitol syrup once per day and a sorbitol syrup twice a day. While more than half of the children in the control group had tooth decay after 10 months, there were significantly fewer caries in both of the xylitol groups. The authors concluded that providing xylitol syrup to infants at least twice a day could reduce early childhood decay by over 70 percent. Fortunately, parents can get these same results thanks to the development of a commercial xylitol tooth gel under the Spry brand that contains calcium and can be delivered through a clever "time release" pacifier.

Another study found that preschoolers who chewed a xylitol gum three times daily for three weeks greatly reduced the amount of S. mutans bacteria in their saliva. A third trial of elementary school students in Washington state noted that those who ate xylitol sweetened gummy bears at school three times a day had a marked reduction in bacteria after just six weeks.

Mixed dentition is a time, generally between ages 5 and 12, when both baby teeth and adult teeth are present. This is another critical time because adult teeth that erupt into a clean xylitol environment are likely to have long-lasting protection against tooth decay.

While there is no doubt that xylitol gum and candy is a tasty and effective way to boost a child's dental health, many parents may wonder if it's safe for very young children. In the amounts recommended—from 5 to 8 grams, or about a heaping teaspoon—xylitol is extremely safe for children of all ages. Most of the xylitol research studies have been conducted on children. It's so safe that, according to Professor Mäkinen, even premature infants possess full capacity to metabolize xylitol. And don't worry about encouraging a "sweet tooth." Preference for sweet taste is innate and was likely a survival advantage for our ancestors.

Smart Snacking

Brushing, flossing, and rinsing can go a long way toward ensuring oral health, especially if you use products containing xylitol. But, to get the optimum health benefits from this natural sweetener, it's also wise to supplement your oral hygiene program with xylitol gum, mints, and candy. Since the ideal exposure is five times daily, enjoying these beneficial snacks between meals can add an additional layer of protection throughout the day.

Study after study shows that chewing xylitol gum decreases the acidity of both saliva and plaque. Researchers have found that this not only lowers S. mutans counts, it also reduces the "stickiness" of plaque so it doesn't readily adhere to teeth. Routinely chewing xylitol gum also encourages remineralization. Sucking on xylitol mints or candies can have a similar effect. Xylitol is most effective when you suck or chew it after eating since this offers both quick and prolonged defense. This makes xylitol gum and candy the ideal delivery system.

Just be aware that some products contain only "token" amounts of xylitol—enough so that they can list it on the package, but not enough to prevent tooth decay. Whether you are shopping for a xylitol toothpaste, mouthwash or pack of gum, look for a product that lists xylitol as the first ingredient, or at least the first—and only—sweetener.

Chapter Four

Xylitol's Other Health Benefits

As you've seen, xylitol plays an important role in dental health. But there's more to this sweetener than simply protecting your pearly whites. Research conducted in more than 40 countries around the world has shown that xylitol promotes upper-respiratory health, supports weight loss, increases bone density, and helps to stabilize blood sugar in people with diabetes and hypoglycemia.

Upper-Respiratory Health

Xylitol can help prevent middle ear infections (otitis media) in children by preventing the growth of bacteria in the tubes that connect the nose and ear. Since about half of all babies suffer from at least one painful ear infection during their first year of life, this is great news for parents. When researchers from the University of Oulu in Finland exposed 159 infants and toddlers to xylitol syrup five times a day, they found that the sweetener cut the number of ear infections by 30 percent. But these benefits aren't just reserved for the very young. Two studies of more than 1,000 pre-kindergarteners show that chewing xylitol gum five times a day can lower bacterial levels and decrease the number of ear infections by 40 percent.

These results prompted Dr. Lon Jones to add xylitol to a saline nasal spray as a superior delivery system for the upper respiratory tract. The xylitol/saline spray worked so well for his granddaughter that he expanded use into his practice with remarkable results. Patients using his spray had fewer ear and sinus infections, along with reports of relief from asthma and allergy symptoms.

One of the primary ways bacteria enter the body is through the nose and mouth, where they attach themselves to mucous membranes. When *Streptococcus pneumoniae* and other harmful bacteria make their home in the upper respiratory passages, they multiply—and this population boom can lead to upper respiratory infection and disease. Xylitol, when used in either a nasal spray or nasal wash, prevents bacteria from sticking to the nasal passages and helps the body remove them, reducing the risk of infection.

Using a xylitol nasal spray regularly also hydrates the nasal passages and helps flush out airborne pollutants that can trigger asthma and allergies. It can also help shrink swollen membranes to allow easy nasal breathing, which is important for developing dental arches in growing children.

Insulin Resistance And Diabetes

Diabetes. If you don't have it, you probably know someone who does. Type 2 diabetes—also known as adult-onset diabetes—has become an epidemic in the United States. More than 20 million Americans suffer from the disease. More frightening still, type 2 diabetes, once rare among people under the age of 20, is being diagnosed more frequently in children and teens.

Diabetes usually begins as insulin resistance, a disorder in which the cells don't use insulin properly. As the need for insulin rises, the pancreas gradually loses its ability to produce it. What triggers this insulin dilemma? Scientists have linked insulin resistance with aging, a family history of diabetes, high amounts of fructose consumption, impaired glucose metabolism, or a sedentary lifestyle. It's more common than you think: Nearly one-third of Americans have insulin resistance, and the number is growing.

People suffering from either of these conditions are sensitive to foods with a high glycemic index. The glycemic index (GI) is a rating scale used to indicate how quickly a particular food raises blood sugar. The higher the number, the faster the rise. Refined white sugar, for instance, has a GI of 85. Xylitol, on the other hand, has a GI of just 7. This means that xylitol is absorbed more slowly than sugar, so it does not contribute to a rapid spike in blood sugar levels or the resulting hyperglycemia caused by an insufficient insulin response.

Several studies have found that, since xylitol consumption doesn't increase blood sugar levels, it is an excellent tool for diabetics looking for tasty and convenient ways to control their blood glucose levels. And since it can be measured cup for cup just like sugar, it's a useful bulk sweetener for anyone with diabetes or insulin resistance.

Weight Control

Not only is xylitol low on the glycemic index, it's also low in calories. Xylitol contains 2.4 calories per gram compared to sugar's 4 calories per gram. This makes it a nice sugar substitute for those trying to lose weight.

Because xylitol is slowly and incompletely absorbed and metabolized in the body, it also acts much like soluble dietary fiber, improving gut health and increasing satiety. This helps you feel full longer after eating. There is preliminary evidence suggesting that xylitol can curb your cravings for

Refined white sugar, for instance, has a GI of 85. Xylitol, on the other hand, has a GI of just 7.

carbohydrates and sweets. As a bonus, xylitol doesn't have any unpleasant aftertaste like many sugar substitutes on the market.

Bone Health

Most of us take our bones for granted, at least until we are older. But the truth is that bone mass begins to decline as early as our mid-30s, making us vulnerable to osteoporosis in our 60s, 70s, and beyond. The statistics for osteoporosis are truly astounding. According to the National Osteoporosis Foundation, osteoporosis threatens an estimated 44 million Americans—or 55 percent of people over the age of 50. Eighty percent of these are women.

Osteoporosis, which literally means "porous bones," is a disease in which the bones gradually lose their density and begin to deteriorate. As a result, bones become brittle and highly susceptible to fractures. This is a significant cause of crippling disability and death in the aged. Many elderly people who suffer a hip fracture lose the ability to walk. Most significantly, up to 36 percent of people who have broken a hip die within one year from complications. Another one-third never regained the ability to function on their own. These people spend the rest of their lives requiring long-term care in nursing facilities.

While calcium has taken center-stage when it comes to the prevention of osteoporosis, xylitol may well be an unsung hero of bone health. Xylitol has been shown to increase calcium absorption in both the small and the large intestines. If the body is able to better use the calcium it receives, the loss of bone density may be slowed. Animal studies suggest that calcium combined with xylitol may also help the body form new bone mineral.

Skin Health

Bones aren't the only things that break down as we age. Skin also begins losing its structural support as the years pass. While hundreds of expensive lotions and potions promise to reverse this structural breakdown, simply adding xylitol to your daily routine may help preserve the skin's integrity and maintain moisture.

Skin is your body's largest organ and is a barrier against the elements. One of the main components that keeps skin structurally strong and healthy is a fibrous protein called collagen. Research indicates that consuming xylitol on a regular basis increases skin thickness and collagen content. In one study, scientists found that xylitol not only spurs the synthesis of new collagen, it also slows down the deterioration of the collagen you already have.

Xylitol may also help skin plagued by the *Staphylococcus aureus* bacteria, a condition known as atopic dermatitis. The most typical symptom of atopic dermatitis is excessively dry skin and a red, itchy rash. Skin creams that contain xylitol have been shown to ease atopic dermatitis by reducing levels of this bacteria and increasing the moisture content of skin.

The anti-biofilm effects of xylitol may be useful in certain topical wound-healing situations. Therapy that includes xylitol has shown promise in the treatment of diabetic ulcers.

Final Thoughts

I've been using xylitol—and recommending it to my patients—for more than 20 years, with wonderful results. Over the years, xylitol has proven its ability to thwart tooth decay and enhance overall dental health in both children and adults.

Adopting a daily dental care routine that includes safe, natural xylitol products is one of the best preventative steps you can take for a healthy mouth. It's also one of the easiest. Switching to a xylitol-based toothpaste and mouthwash is a great place to start. Adding chewing gum, mints, and other xylitol treats adds even more protection—and it's a delicious way to keep dental caries and gum disease at bay.

Emerging research also suggests that xylitol offers a number of other health benefits, from helping control blood sugar to enhancing respiratory health and building stronger bones. As science discovers more ways that xylitol can improve our health, you are sure to see it appear in an ever-increasing number of products.

For now, xylitol's remarkable dental benefits and safety record make it an ideal addition to a healthy lifestyle. The xylitol plan is simple: Morning and night, brush with xylitol toothpaste, floss, rinse with xylitol mouthwash, and spray with xylitol/saline nasal spray. After meals and snacks, use at least one piece of xylitol gum or candy.

I urge you to give it a try. I'm sure that once you experience xylitol's benefits for yourself, you will have something very sweet to smile about.

Glossary

Abscess: Infected, pus-filled, inflamed area around a tooth.

Acid: Corrosive compound produced during the bacterial conversion of food, especially sugars and starches.

Alveolar bone: The specialized bony structure that supports the teeth; it consists of the cortical bone that comprises the tooth socket into which the roots of the tooth fit, and is supported by the trabecular bone.

Caries: Progressive demineralization by microbial acids leading to destruction or necrosis of teeth.

Cavity: Hole in the tooth caused by the caries process.

Cementum: A layer of bone-like mineralized tissue that covers the roots of a tooth.

Decay: Destruction of teeth by caries.

Demineralization: A loss of the mineral constituents of the teeth or alveolar bone.

Dentin: The hard, living inner layer of a tooth (the layer immediately under the outer enamel layer).

Enamel: The hardest, most highly mineralized substance of the body, covering the dentin and forming the outer layer of the tooth.

Fluoride: A mineral added to toothpaste and drinking water that can strengthen and repair the surface of teeth and prevent caries.

Gingiva: The soft tissue that surrounds the base of the teeth. Commonly called the gums.

Gingivitis: Inflammation of the gingiva in response to bacterial plaque on adjacent teeth.

Halitosis: The clinical term for bad breath.

Hard Palate: The bony part of the roof of the mouth.

Impaction: A tooth that is not able to come in normally or is stuck underneath another tooth or bone.

Mandible: The U-shaped bone that forms the lower jaw and holds the lower teeth in place.

Maxilla: Either of the two bones that together form the upper jaw and support the upper teeth.

Periodontitis: An inflammatory disease of the supporting structures that hold the teeth in place, characterized by deepening gum pockets and loss of alveolar bone.

Plaque: A biofilm of bacteria in a sticky matrix that adheres to the teeth that encourages the development of dental caries and periodontal disease.

Polyols: Sugars that have been "reduced" by the addition of hydrogen. Also known as sugar alcohols, polyols are not completely absorbed and metabolized by the body. Because of this, polyols contribute fewer calories than other natural bulk sweeteners.

Pulp: The soft tissue in the center of the tooth that contains nerves, blood vessels, and connective tissue.

Remineralization: In dentistry, a process whereby partially decalcified enamel, dentin, and cementum become recalcified by mineral replacement.

Soft Palate: The soft tissue constituting the back of the roof of the mouth.

***Streptococcus mutans*:** A group of acid-tolerant, acid-producing, cariogenic (decay-causing) oral bacteria that includes *Streptococcus mutans* and *Streptococcus sobrinus.*

Tartar: A hardened white, brown, or yellow-brown deposit at or below the gumline of teeth. Also called calculus.

Selected References

Ahluwalia KP. Oral disease experience of older adults seeking oral health services. *Gerodontology*. Sep 8 2009.

Berman JR. Physiology of female sexual function and dysfunction. *International Journal of Impotence Research*. 17 Suppl 1:S44-51, 2005.

Biesbrock A. Assessment of Treatment Responses to Dental Flossing in Twins. *Journal of Periodontology*. 77; 1386-1391, 2006.

Buencamino MC. How menopause affects oral health, and what we can do about it. *Cleveland Clinic Journal of Medicine*. 76:467-475, 2009.

Coldwell SE. A marker of growth differs between adolescents with high vs. low sugar preference. *Physiology and Behavior*. 96:574-580, 2009.

Fitzpatrick SG. The Association Between Periodontal Disease and Cancer: A Review of the Literature. *Journal of Dentistry*. 2009 Nov 3.

Haumschild MS. The importance of oral health in long-term care. *Journal of the American Medical Directors Association*. 10:667-671, 2009.

Holgerson PL. Dental plaque formation and salivary mutans streptococci in schoolchildren after use of xylitol-containing chewing gum. *International Journal of Paediatric Dentistry*. 17:79-85, 2007.

Jimenez M. Periodontitis and incidence of cerebrovascular disease in men. *Annals of Neurology*. 66:505-512, 2009.

Katsuyama M. A novel method to control the balance of skin microflora Part 2. A study to assess the effect of a cream containing farnesol and xylitol on atopic dry skin. *Journal of Dermatological Science*. 38:207-213, 2005.

Khovidhunkit SO. Xerostomia, hyposalivation, and oral microbiota in type 2 diabetic patients: a preliminary study. *Journal of the Medical Assocication of Thailand*. 92:1220-1228, 2009.

King NA. Evaluation of the independent and combined effects of xylitol and polydextrose consumed as a snack on hunger and energy intake over 10 d. *British Journal of Nutrition*. 93:911-915, 2005.

Lif Holgerson P. Xylitol Concentration in Saliva and Dental Plaque after Use of Various Xylitol-Containing Products. *Caries Research*. 40:393-397, 2006.

Ly KA. Xylitol gummy bear snacks: a school-based randomized clinical trial. *BMC Oral Health*. 8:20, 2008.

Ly KA. Xylitol, sweeteners, and dental caries. *Pediatric Dentistry*. 28:154-163, 2006.

Mäkinen KK. Thirty-nine-month xylitol chewing-gum programme in initially 8-year-old school children: a feasibility study focusing on mutans streptococci and lactobacilli. *International Dental Journal*. 58:41-50, 2008.

Mäkinen KK. *Xylitol: An Amazing Discovery for Health*. Woodland Publishing, Orem, UT. 2007.

Mattila PT. Effects of a long-term dietary xylitol supplementation on collagen content and fluorescence of the skin in aged rats. *Gerontology*. 51:166-169, 2005.

Mattila PT. The effect of a simultaneous dietary administration of xylitol and ethanol on bone resorption. *Metabolism*. 54:548-551, 2005.

Milgrom P. Mutans streptococci dose response to xylitol chewing gum. *Journal of Dental Research*. 85:177-181, 2006.

Milgrom P. Xylitol pediatric topical oral syrup to prevent dental caries: a double-blind randomized clinical trial of efficacy. *Archives of Pediatrics & Adolescent Medicine*. 163:601-607, 2009.

Nakai Y. Influence of maternal xylitol consumption on mother-child transmission of cariogenic bacteria during and after pregnancy. *Finnish Dental Journal*. 1:12-17, 2006.

Natah SS. Metabolic Response to Lactitol and Xylitol in Healthy Men, *American Journal of Clinical Nutrition* 65:947-950, 1997.

Oral Health: Preventing Cavities, Gum Disease, and Tooth Loss. U.S. Department of Health and Human Services. Centers for Disease Control and Prevention. Coodinating Center for Health Promotion. 2007.

Patiño Marín N. Caries, periodontal disease and tooth loss in patients with diabetes mellitus types 1 and 2. Acta *Odontológica Latinoamericana*. 21:127-133, 2008.

Sano H. Effect of a xylitol and fluoride containing toothpaste on the remineralization of human enamel in vitro. *Journal of Oral Science*. 49:67-73, 2007.

Söderling E. Xylitol reduces mother-child transmission of mutans streptococci. *Finnish Dental Journal*. 1:8-11, 2006.

Splieth CH. Effect of xylitol and sorbitol on plaque acidogenesis. *Quintessence International*. 40:279-285, 2009.

Tezal M. Periodontal disease and the incidence of tooth loss in postmenopausal women. *Journal of Periodontology*. 76:1123-1128, 2005.

Thaweboon S. Remineralization of enamel subsurface lesions by xylitol chewing gum containing funoran and calcium hydrogenphosphate. *Southeast Asian Journal of Tropical Medicine and Public Health*. 40:345-353, 2009.

Trends in Oral Health Status: United States, 1988–1994 and 1999–2004. Data From the Continuous National Health and Nutrition Examination Survey (NHANES). Vital and Health Statistics, Series 11. U.S. Department of Health and Human Services. Centers for Disease Control and Prevention. National Center for Health Statistics. 2007.

Twetman S. Consistent evidence to support the use of xylitol- and sorbitol-containing chewing gum to prevent dental caries. *Evidence Based Dentistry*. 10:10-11, 2009.

Vouros ID. Cigarette smoking associated with advanced periodontal destruction in a Greek sample population of patients with periodontal disease. *Journal of the International Academy of Periodontology*. 11;250-257, 2009.

Yoshihara A. A longitudinal study of the relationship between diet intake and dental caries and periodontal disease in elderly Japanese subjects. *Gerodontology*. 26:130-136, 2009.

Yuan J. The effect of "Oral Wet" for elderly people with xerostomia—the effect of oral rinse containing hialuronan. *Kokubyo Gakkai Zasshi*. 72:106-110, 2005.

For more information on Xlear, Inc., and xylitol-based dental care and respiratory health products, visit www.xlear.com.